LOW CARB COOKBOOK- SOUPS&V

DELICIOUS ,EASY AND LOW BUDGET RECIPES TO RESET YOUR METABOLISM,LOSE WEIGHT FASTER& KEEP THE CORRECT LIFE-STYLE.

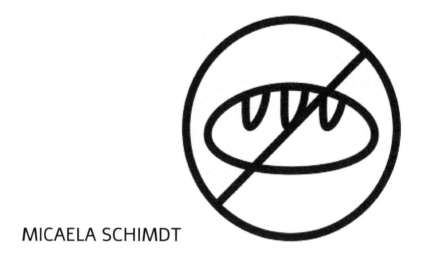

MICAELA SCHIMDT

TABLE OF CONTENTS

Introduction

The LOW-CARB Diet is a high-fat eating regimen, which seems to profit a few people with epilepsy, particularly youngsters. It's anything but an enchantment fix; however, one option in contrast to the different enemy of epileptic drugs at present accessible. The Ketogenic diet offers the benefit of improved seizure control for youngsters, and at times, improved mental sharpness with fewer meds.

The LOW-CARB diet is regularly viewed as a troublesome routine to follow. As it may, with training and an arrangement what the eating regimen plans to accomplish, it very well may be decreased to a sensible everyday practice. The fundamental point is to switch the body's essential fuel source from starches (like bread and sugar) to fats. That is finished by expanding the admission of fats and significantly lessening the admission of starches. The real trouble is that the eating regimen is prohibitive to such an extent that all nourishments eaten must be weighed out to a 10th of a gram during feast Preparing, and a member may not eat anything which is not "endorsed" by the dietician. The degree of starches permitted is deficient so that even the limited quantity of sugar in generally fluid or chewable drugs will keep the eating regimen from working.

As specific illustrations, a commonplace supper may incorporate some meat with green vegetables cooked with a mayonnaise sauce or a great deal of margarine. Weighty cream might be remembered for the side for drinking. Another dinner may comprise of bacon and eggs with a great deal of margarine or oil added and heavy cream to drink. A too high proportion of fats to sugars must be kept up with a low all out calorie consumption for the eating regimen to be fruitful.

BENEFITS OF LOW CARB DIET

There are reliable and keto bites that can top you off on the off chance that you get ravenous between suppers. They incorporate a couple of hard-bubbled eggs, infant carrots with a tablespoon or two of a LOW-CARB plunging sauce, full-fat yogurt with a tablespoon, or two new berries, a small bunch of nuts, and a couple of cheddar sticks.

1. Supports weight reduction

The LOW CARB diet may help advance weight reduction in a few different ways, including boosting digestion and decreasing hunger.

LOW-CARB eats less comprise of nourishments that top an individual off and may diminish hunger-invigorating hormones. Therefore, following a LOW CARB diet may diminish craving and advance weight reduction.

Likewise, another audit of 11 studies showed that individuals following a LOW-CARB diet lost 5 lbs more than those after low-fat eating regimens following a half year.

1. Improves skin break out

Skin break out has a few unique causes and may have connections to abstain from food and glucose in specific individuals.

Eating an eating regimen high in handled and refined starches may adjust the equilibrium of gut microorganisms and cause glucose to rise and fall practice, the two of which can antagonistically influence skin well-being.

By diminishing carb admission, a LOW-CARB diet could lessen skin inflammation indications in specific individuals.

1. May diminish the danger of specific malignant growths.

Analysts have analyzed the impacts of the LOW-CARB diet in forestalling or even treat certain diseases.

One study found that the LOW-CARB diet might be a sheltered and appropriate integral therapy to use close by chemotherapy and radiation treatment in individuals with specific tumors. It would cause more oxidative pressure in disease cells than in typical cells, making them pass on.

A later report from 2018 recommends that because the LOW-CARB diet diminishes glucose, it could bring down the danger of insulin entanglements. Insulin is a hormone that controls glucose that may have connections to certain malignant growths.

Although some examination demonstrates that the LOW-CARB diet may have some advantages in disease treatment, concentrates here are restricted.

1. May improve heart well-being.

When an individual follows the LOW CARB diet, it is significant that they pick energizing nourishments. Some proof shows that eating refreshing fats and avocados rather than less energizing fats, such as pork skins, can help improve heart well-being by decreasing cholesterol.

A 2017 survey of investigations of creatures and people on a LOW-CARB diet demonstrated that a few people encountered a massive drop in levels of all-out cholesterol, low-thickness lipoprotein (LDL), or terrible cholesterol, and fatty substances, and an expansion in high-thickness lipoprotein (HDL), or "great" cholesterol.

Significant levels of cholesterol can expand the danger of cardiovascular infection. A LOW-CARB diet's decreasing impact on cholesterol may, like this, diminish an individual's danger of heart confusion. Nonetheless, the survey reasoned that the eating routine's beneficial outcomes on heart well-being rely upon diet quality. In this way, it is essential to eat empowering, healthfully adjusted food while following the LOW-CARB diet.

Stunning Broccoli and Cauliflower Cream

That is so finished and flavorful!

Preparing time: 10 min Time for cooking: 15 min Platefuls: 5

Ingredients:
- One cauliflower head, florets isolated
- One broccoli head, florets isolated
- Salt and dark pepper to the taste
- Two garlic cloves, minced
- Two bacon slices, sliced

- Two tablespoons ghee

Directions:

1. Warmth up a pot with the ghee over medium-high warmth, include garlic and bacon, mix and cook for 3 min.

2. Include cauliflower and broccoli florets, mix, and cook for 2 min more.

3. Add water to cover them, spread the pot, and stew for 10 min.

4. Place salt and pepper, mix again, and mix soup utilizing a drenching blender.

5. Stew for a couple more min over medium warmth, scoop into bowls, and serve.

Relax and enjoy!

Nourishment: calories 230, fat 3, fiber 3, carbs 6, protein 10

Broccoli Stew

This veggie stew is merely tasty!

Preparing time: 10 min Time for cooking: 40 min Platefuls: 4

Ingredients:

- One broccoli head, florets isolated

- Two teaspoons coriander seeds
- A shower of olive oil
- One yellow onion, sliced
- Salt and dark pepper to the taste
- A touch of red pepper squashed
- One little ginger piece, sliced
- One garlic clove, minced
- 28 ounces canned tomatoes, pureed

Directions:

1. Pour water inside a clean pot, place salt, heat to the point of boiling over medium-high warmth, include broccoli florets, steam them for 2 min, move them to a bowl loaded up with ice water, channel them and leave aside.

2. Warmth up a skillet over medium-high warmth, include coriander seeds, toast them for 4 min, move to a processor, ground them, and leave aside.

3. Warmth up a pot with the oil over medium warmth, include onions, salt, pepper, and red pepper, mix and cook for 7 min.

4. Include ginger, garlic, and coriander seeds, mix, and cook for 3 min.

5. Include tomatoes, heat to the point of boiling, and stew for 10 min.

6. Include broccoli; mix and cook your stew for 12 min.

7. Partition into bowls and serve.

Relax and enjoy!

Nourishment: calories 150, fat 4, fiber 2, carbs 5, protein 12

Astounding Watercress Soup

A Chinese style LOW-CARB soup sounds genuinely stunning, isn't that right?

Preparing time: 10 min Time for cooking: 10 min Platefuls: 4

Ingredients:

- 6 cup chicken stock

- ¼ cup sherry

- Two teaspoons coconut amino

- Six and ½ cups watercress

- Salt and dark pepper to the taste
- Two teaspoons sesame seed
- Three shallots, sliced
- Three egg whites whisked

Directions:

1. Put the stock into a pot, blend in with salt, pepper, sherry, and coconut amino, mix and heat to the point of boiling over medium-high warmth.

2. Include shallots, watercress, egg whites, mix, heat to the point of boiling, partition into bowls, and present with sesame seeds sprinkled on top.

Relax and enjoy!

Nourishment: calories 50, fat 1, fiber 0, carbs 1, protein 5

Heavenly Bok Choy Soup

You can even have this for supper!

Preparing time: 10 min Time for cooking: 15 min Platefuls: 4

Ingredients:

- 3 cups hamburger stock
- One yellow onion, sliced
- One bundle bok choy, sliced
- One and ½ cups mushrooms, sliced
- Salt and dark pepper to the taste
- ½ tablespoon red pepper drops
- Three tablespoons coconut amino
- Three tablespoons parmesan, ground
- Two tablespoons Worcestershire sauce
- Two bacon strips, sliced

Directions:
1. Warmth up a pot over medium-high warmth, include bacon, mix, cook until it's fresh, move to paper towels and channel oil.
2. Warmth up the pot again over medium warmth, include mushrooms and onions, mix and cook for 5 min.
3. Include stock, bok choy, coconut amino, salt, pepper, pepper drops, and Worcestershire sauce, mix, spread, and cook until bok choy is delicate.

4. Spoon soup into bowls, sprinkle parmesan and bacon, and serve.

Relax and enjoy!

Nourishment: calories 100, fat 3, fiber 1, carbs 2, protein 6

Bok Choy Stir Fry

It's straightforward; it's simple and tasty!

Preparing time: 10 min Time for cooking: 7 min Platefuls: 2

Ingredients:

- Two garlic cloves, minced

- 2 cup bok choy, sliced

- Two bacon slices, sliced

- Salt and dark pepper to the taste

- A shower of avocado oil

Directions:

1. Warmth up a dish with the oil over medium warmth, include bacon, mix and earthy colored until it's firm, move to paper towels and channel oil.

2. Return dish to medium warmth, include garlic and bok choy, mix and cook for 4 min.
3. Place salt, pepper and return bacon, mix, cook for brief more, separate among plates, and serve.
Relax and enjoy!
Nourishment: calories 50, fat 1, fiber 1, carbs 2, protein 2

Cream of Celery

That will dazzle you!
Preparing time: 10 min Time for cooking: 40 min Platefuls: 4
Ingredients:

- One pack celery, sliced
- Salt and dark pepper to the taste
- Three straight leaves
- ½ garlic head, sliced
- Two yellow onions, sliced
- 4 cups chicken stock
- ¾ cup hefty cream

- Two tablespoons ghee

Directions:
1. Warmth up a pot with the ghee over medium-high warmth, include onions, salt, and pepper, mix and cook for 5 min.
2. Include straight leaves, garlic, and celery, mix, and cook for 15 min.
3. Include stock, salt, pepper, mix, spread pot, diminish warmth, and stew for 20 min.
4. Include cream, mix, and mix everything utilizing a drenching blender.
5. Scoop into soup bowls and serve.
Relax and enjoy!
Nourishment: calories 150, fat 3, fiber 1, carbs 2, protein 6

Awesome Celery Soup

It's so awesome and heavenly! Attempt it!
Preparing time: 10 min Time for cooking: 25 min Platefuls: 8
Ingredients:
- 26 ounces celery leaves and stems, sliced

- One tablespoon onion drops

- Salt and dark pepper to the taste

- Three teaspoons fenugreek powder
- Three teaspoons veggie stock powder
- 10 ounces harsh cream

Directions:

1. Put celery into a pot, add water to cover, include onion drops, salt, pepper, stock powder, and fenugreek powder, mix, heat to the point of boiling over medium warmth stew for 20 min.

2. Utilize a submersion blender to make your cream; include acrid cream, more salt and pepper, and mix once more.

3. Warmth up soup again over medium warmth, scoop into bowls and serve.

Relax and enjoy!

Nourishment: calories 140, fat 2, fiber 1, carbs 5, protein 10

Stunning Celery Stew

This Iranian style Keto stew is so delicious and simple to make!

Preparing time: 10 min Time for cooking: 30 min Platefuls: 6

Ingredients:

- One celery bundle, generally sliced
- One yellow onion, sliced
- One bundle green onion, sliced
- Four garlic cloves, minced
- Salt and dark pepper to the taste
- One parsley bundle, sliced
- Two mint bundles, sliced
- Three dried Persian lemons, pricked with a fork
- 2 cups of water
- Two teaspoons chicken bouillon
- Four tablespoons olive oil

Directions:
1. Warmth up a pot with the oil over medium-high warmth, include onion, green onions, and garlic, mix and cook for 6 min.
2. Include celery, Persian lemons, chicken bouillon, salt, pepper, water, mix, spread pot, and stew on medium warmth for 20 min.
3. Include parsley and mint; mix and cook for 10 min more.

4. Separation into bowls and serve.
Relax and enjoy!
Nourishment: calories 170, fat 7, fiber 4, carbs 6, protein 10

Spinach Soup

It's a finished and smooth Keto soup you need to attempt soon!
Preparing time: 10 min Time for cooking: 15 min Platefuls: 8

Ingredients:

- Two tablespoons ghee

- 20 ounces spinach, sliced

- One teaspoon garlic, minced

- Salt and dark pepper to the taste

- 45 ounces chicken stock

- ½ teaspoon nutmeg, ground

- 2 cups substantial cream

- One yellow onion, sliced

Directions:

1. Warmth up a pot with the ghee over medium warmth, include onion, mix and cook for 4 min.
2. Include garlic, mix, and cook for one moment.
3. Include spinach and stock, mix, and cook for 5 min.
4. Mix soup with an inundation blender and warmth up the soup once more.
5. Place salt, pepper, nutmeg, and cream, mix and cook for 5 min more.
6. Spoon into bowls and serve.
Relax and enjoy!
Nourishment: calories 245, fat 24, fiber 3, carbs 4, protein 6

Delightful Mustard Greens Sauté

That is so delectable!
Preparing time: 10 min Time for cooking: 20 min Platefuls: 4
Ingredients:

- Two garlic cloves, minced

- One tablespoon olive oil

- Two and ½ pounds collard greens, sliced
- One teaspoon lemon juice
- One tablespoon ghee
- Salt and dark pepper to the taste

Directions:
1. Pour some water in a pot, add salt, and bring a stew over medium warmth.
2. Include greens, spread, and cook for 15 min.
3. Channel collard greens well, press out fluid, and put them into a bowl.
4. Warmth up a dish with the oil and the ghee over medium-high warmth, including collard greens, salt, pepper, and garlic.
5. Mix well and cook for 5 min.
6. Include more salt and pepper if necessary, shower lemon juice, mix, partition among plates, and serve.
Relax and enjoy!
Nourishment: calories 151, fat 6, fiber 3, carbs 7, protein 8

Scrumptious Collards Greens and Ham

This delicious dish will be prepared in no time! Preparing time: 10 min Time for cooking: 1 hour and 40 min Platefuls: 4

Ingredients:

- 4 ounces ham, boneless, cooked and sliced

- One tablespoon olive oil

- 2 pounds collard greens, cut into medium strips

- One teaspoon red pepper chips, squashed

- Salt and dark pepper to the taste

- 2 cups chicken stock

- One yellow onion, sliced

- 4 ounces dry white wine

- 1-ounce salt pork

- ¼ cup apple juice vinegar

- ½ cup ghee, dissolved

Directions:

1. Warmth up a dish with the oil over medium-high warmth, include ham and onion, mix and cook for 4 min.

2. Place salt pork, collard greens, stock, vinegar, and wine, mix, and heat to the point of boiling.

3. Decrease heat, spread skillet, and cook for 1 hour and 30 min blending occasionally.

4. Include ghee, dispose of salt pork, mix, cook everything for 10 min, separate among plates, and serve.

Relax and enjoy!

Nourishment: calories 150, fat 12, fiber 2, carbs 4, protein 8

Delicious Collard Greens and Tomatoes

That is simply phenomenal!

Preparing time: 10 min Time for cooking: 12 min Platefuls:5

Ingredients:

- 1 pound collard greens

- Three bacon strips, sliced

- ¼ cup cherry tomatoes split
- One tablespoon apple juice vinegar
- Two tablespoons chicken stock
- Salt and dark pepper to the taste

Directions:

1. Warmth up a dish over medium warmth, include bacon, mix and cook until it earthy colors.

2. Include tomatoes, collard greens, vinegar, stock, salt, pepper, mix, and cook for 8 min.

3. Include more salt and pepper, mix again tenderly, isolate among plates, and serve. Relax and enjoy!

Nourishment: calories 120, fat 8, fiber 1, carbs 3, protein 7

Basic Mustard Greens Dish

Everybody can make this basic Keto dish! You'll see!

Preparing time: 5 min Time for cooking: 15 min Platefuls: 4

Ingredients:

- Two garlic cloves, minced

- 1 pound mustard greens, torn
- One tablespoon olive oil
- ½ cup yellow onion, sliced
- Salt and dark pepper to the taste
- Three tablespoons veggie stock
- ¼ teaspoon dull sesame oil

Directions:

1. Warmth up a dish with the oil over medium warmth, include onions, mix, and earthy colored them for 10 min.

2. Include garlic, mix, and cook for one moment.

3. Include stock, greens, salt, pepper, mix, and cook for 5 min more.

4. Include more salt and pepper and the sesame oil, throw to cover, separate among plates, and serve.

Relax and enjoy!

Nourishment: calories 120, fat 3, fiber 1, carbs 3, protein 6

Tasty Collard Greens and Poached Eggs

That will genuinely make everybody love your cooking!

Preparing time: 10 min Time for cooking: 15 min Platefuls: 6

Ingredients:

- One tablespoon chipotle in adobo pounded

- Six eggs

- Three tablespoons ghee

- One yellow onion, sliced

- Two garlic cloves, minced

- Six bacon slices, sliced

- Three bundles collard greens, sliced

- ½ cup chicken stock

- Salt and dark pepper to the taste

- One tablespoon lime juice

- Some ground cheddar

Directions:

1. Warmth up a skillet over medium-high warmth, include bacon, cook until it's fresh, move to paper towels, channel oil, and leave aside.

2. Warmth up the skillet again over medium warmth, include garlic and onion, mix and cook for 2 min.

3. Return bacon to the skillet, mix and cook for 3 min more.

4. Include chipotle in adobo glue, collard greens, salt, pepper, mix, and cook for 10 min.

5. Include stock and lime squeeze and mix.

6. Make six gaps in collard greens blend, isolate ghee in them, break an egg in each gap, spread dish, and cook until eggs are finished.

7. Partition this among plates and present with cheddar sprinkled on top.

Relax and enjoy!

Nourishment: calories 245, fat 20, fiber 1, carbs 5, protein 12

Collard Greens Soup

That is a Keto soup even vegans will adore!

Preparing time: 10 min Time for cooking: 40 min Platefuls: 12

Ingredients:

- One teaspoon bean stew powder
- One tablespoon avocado oil
- Two teaspoons smoked paprika
- One teaspoon cumin
- One yellow onion, sliced
- A spot of red pepper drops
- 10 cups water
- Three celery stems, sliced
- Three carrots, sliced
- 15 ounces canned tomatoes, sliced
- Two tablespoons tamari sauce
- 6 ounces canned tomato glue
- Two tablespoons lemon juice
- Salt and dark pepper to the taste
- 6 cups collard greens, stems disposed of
- One tablespoon turn
- One teaspoon garlic granules
- One tablespoon spice preparing

Directions:

1. Warmth up a pot with the oil over medium-high warmth, include cumin, pepper drops, paprika, and bean stew powder, and mix well.

2. Include celery, onion, and carrots, mix, and cook for 10 min.

3. Include tamari sauce, tomatoes, tomato glue, water, lemon juice, salt, pepper, spice preparing, turn, garlic granules, and collard greens, mix, heat to the point of boiling, spread, and cook for 30 min.

4. Mix once more, spoon into bowls and serve. Relax and enjoy!

Nourishment: calories 150, fat 3, fiber 2, carbs 4, protein 8

Spring Green Soup

That is a crisp spring Ketogenic soup! Preparing time: 10 min Time for cooking: 30 min Platefuls: 4

Ingredients:

- 2 cups mustard greens, sliced

- 2 cups collard greens, sliced

- 3 quarts veggie stock

- One yellow onion, sliced
- Salt and dark pepper to the taste
- Two tablespoons coconut amino
- Two teaspoons ginger, ground

Directions:

1. Place the stock into a pot and bring to a stew over medium-high warmth.

2. Include mustard and collard greens, onion, salt, pepper, coconut amino, ginger, mix, spread pot, and cook for 30 min.

3. Mix soup utilizing an inundation blender, include more salt and pepper, heat up over medium warmth, scoop into soup bowls, and serve.

Relax and enjoy!

Nourishment: calories 140, fat 2, fiber 1, carbs 3, protein 7

Mustard Greens and Spinach Soup

This Indian style Keto soup is astonishing!
Preparing time: 10 min Time for cooking: 15 min Platefuls: 6

Ingredients:

- ½ teaspoon fenugreek seeds
- One teaspoon cumin seeds
- One tablespoon avocado oil
- One teaspoon coriander seeds
- 1 cup yellow onion, sliced
- One tablespoon garlic, minced
- One tablespoon ginger, ground
- ½ teaspoon turmeric, ground
- 5 cups mustard greens, sliced
- 3 cups of coconut milk
- One tablespoon jalapeno, sliced
- 5 cups spinach, torn
- Salt and dark pepper to the taste
- Two teaspoons ghee
- ½ teaspoon paprika

Directions:

1. Warmth up a pot with the oil over medium-high warmth, include coriander, fenugreek,

and cumin seeds, mix and earthy colored them for 2 min.

2. Include onions, mix, and cook for 3 min more.

3. Include half of the garlic, jalapenos, ginger, and turmeric, mix and cook for 3 min more.

4. Include mustard greens and spinach, mix and sauté everything for 10 min.

5. Include milk, salt, and pepper, and mix soup utilizing a drenching blender.

6. Warmth up a skillet with the ghee over medium warmth, include garlic and paprika, mix well, and take off warmth.

7. Warmth up the soup over medium warmth, scoop into soup bowls, shower ghee, and paprika all finished and soup.

Relax and enjoy!

Nourishment: calories 143, fat 6, fiber 3, carbs 7, protein 7

Broiled Asparagus

It's unbelievably simple and very flavorful!
Preparing time: 10 min Time for cooking: 10 min Platefuls: 3

Ingredients:

- One asparagus pack, managed
- Three teaspoons avocado oil
- A sprinkle of lemon juice
- Salt and dark pepper to the taste
- One tablespoon oregano, sliced

Directions:

1. Spread asparagus lances on a lined preparing sheet, sprinkle with salt and pepper, shower oil and lemon juice, sprinkle oregano, and throw to cover well.

2. Present in the stove at 425 degrees F and prepare for 10 min.

Separation among plates and serve.

Relax and enjoy!

Nourishment: calories 130, fat 1, fiber 1, carbs 2, protein 3

Straightforward Asparagus Fries

These will be prepared in just 10 min!

Preparing time: 10 min Time for cooking: 10 min Platefuls: 2

Ingredients:

- ¼ cup parmesan, ground
- 16 asparagus lances, managed
- One egg whisked
- ½ teaspoon onion powder
- 2 ounces of pork skins

Directions:

1. Smash pork skins and put them in a bowl.
2. Include onion powder and cheddar and mix everything.
3. Move asparagus lances in the egg; at that point, dunk them in pork skin blend and orchestrate them all on a lined preparing sheet.
4. Present in the stove at 425 degrees F and prepare for 10 min.
5. Separation among plates and serve them with some acrid cream as an afterthought. Relax and enjoy!

Nourishment: calories 120, fat 2, fiber 2, carbs 5, protein 8

Astonishing Asparagus and Browned Butter

This Keto dish is exceptionally delightful, and it likewise looks superb!

Preparing time: 10 min Time for cooking: 15 min Platefuls: 4

Ingredients:

- 5 ounces spread

- One tablespoon avocado oil

- One and ½ pounds asparagus, managed

- One and ½ tablespoons lemon juice

- A touch of cayenne pepper

- Eight tablespoons acrid cream

- Salt and dark pepper to the taste

- 3 ounces parmesan, ground

- Four eggs

Directions:

1. Warmth up a container with 2 ounces spread over medium-high warmth, including eggs, salt, and pepper; mix and scramble them.

2. Move eggs to a blender, including parmesan, acrid cream, salt, pepper, and cayenne pepper, and mix everything admirably.

3. Warmth up a container with the oil over medium-high warmth, include asparagus, salt, and pepper, broil for a couple of moments, move to a plate, and leave them aside.

4. Warmth up the skillet again with the remainder of the margarine over medium-high warmth, mix until it's earthy colored, take off warmth, include lemon squeeze, and mix well.

5. Warmth up the spread once more, return asparagus, throw to cover, heat up well, and partition between plates.

6. Include mixed eggs top and serve. Relax and enjoy!

Nourishment: calories 160, fat 7, fiber 2, carbs 6, protein 10.

Asparagus Frittata

It's a super delectable!

Cook time: 10 minutes Cooking time: 15 minutes Servings: 4

Ingredients:
- ¼ cup yellow onion, cleaved
- A sprinkle of olive oil
- 1 pound asparagus lances, cut into 1 inch pieces
- Salt and dark pepper to the taste
- 4 eggs, whisked
- 1 cup cheddar, ground

Directions:
1. Warmth up a container with the oil over medium-high warmth, add onions, mix and cook for 3 minutes.
2. Add asparagus, mix, and cook for 6 minutes.
3. Add eggs, mix a piece, and cook for 3 minutes.
4. Add salt, pepper and sprinkle the cheddar present in the broiler; what's more, sear for 3 minutes.
5. Gap frittata among plates and serve.
Relax and enjoy!
Nourishment: calories 200, fat 12, fiber 2, carbs 5, protein 14

Rich Asparagus

It's a vibrant Keto dish you can attempt this evening!

Cook time: 10 minutes Cooking time: 15 minutes Servings: 3

Ingredients:
- 10 ounces asparagus lances, cut into medium pieces and steamed
- Salt and dark pepper to the taste
- 2 tablespoons parmesan, ground
- 1/3 cup Monterey jack cheddar, destroyed
- 2 tablespoons mustard
- 2 ounces cream cheddar
- 1/3 cup substantial cream
- 3 tablespoons bacon, cooked and disintegrated

Directions:
1. Warmth up a dish with mustard, heavy cream, and cream cheddar over medium warmth and mix well.
2. Add Monterey Jack cheddar and parmesan, mix and cook until it dissolves.

3. Add half of the bacon and the asparagus, mix, and cook for 3 minutes.
4. Add the remainder of the bacon, salt, and pepper, mix, cook for 5 minutes, partition among plates, and serve.
Relax and enjoy!
Nourishment: calories 256, fat 23, fiber 2, carbs 5, protein 13

Tasty Fledglings Serving of mixed greens

That is so new and loaded with nutrients! It's superb!

Preparing time: 10 minutes Cooking time: 0 minutes Servings: 4

Ingredients:
- 1 green apple, cored and julienned
- 1 and ½ teaspoons dull sesame oil
- 4 cups hay sprouts
- Salt and dark pepper to the taste
- 1 and ½ teaspoons grapeseed oil
- ¼ cup coconut milk yogurt

• 4 nasturtium leaves
Directions:
1. In a plate of mixed greens, bowl blend grows in with apple and nasturtium.
2. Add salt, pepper, sesame oil, grape seed oil, coconut yogurt, throw to cover, and separate plates.
3. Serve immediately.
Relax and enjoy!
Nourishment: calories 100, fat 3, fiber 1, carbs 2, protein 6

Broiled Radishes

If you don't have the opportunity to prepare an unpredictable supper today, at that point, attempt this formula!
Preparing time: 10 minutes Cooking time: 35 minutes Servings: 2
Ingredients:
• 2 cups radishes, cut in quarters
• Salt and dark pepper to the taste
• 2 tablespoons ghee, softened
• 1 tablespoon chives, slashed
• 1 tablespoon lemon zing
Directions:

1. Spread radishes on a lined heating sheet.
2. Add salt and pepper, chives, lemon zing, and ghee, throw to cover furthermore, prepare in the broiler at 375 degrees F for 35 minutes.
3. Gap among plates and serve.
Relax and enjoy!
Nourishment: calories 122, fat 12, fiber 1, carbs 3, protein 14

Radish Hash Earthy colors

Would you like to figure out how to make this delectable Keto dish? At that point, focus.
 Preparing time: 10 minutes Cooking time: 10 minutes Servings: 4

Ingredients:
- ½ teaspoon onion powder
- 1 pound radishes, destroyed
- ½ teaspoon garlic powder
- Salt and dark pepper to the taste
- 4 eggs
- 1/3 cup parmesan, ground

Directions:

1. In a bowl, blend radishes with salt, pepper, onion and garlic powder, eggs, and parmesan and mix well.
2. Spread this on a lined preparing sheet, present in the broiler at 375 degrees F, and prepare for 10 minutes.
3. Separation hash browns among plates and serve.
Relax and enjoy!
Nourishment: calories 80, fat 5, fiber 2, carbs 5, protein 7

Firm Radishes

It's an incredible Keto thought!
 Cook time: 10 minutes Cooking time: 20 minutes Servings: 4
Ingredients:
• Cooking splash
• 15 radishes, cut
• Salt and dark pepper to the taste
• 1 tablespoon chives, hacked
Directions:

1. Orchestrate radish cuts on a lined heating sheet and splash them with cooking oil.
2. Season with salt and pepper and sprinkle chives, present in the stove at 375 degrees F, and heat for 10 minutes.
3. Flip them and prepare for 10 minutes more.
4. Serve them cold.

Relax and enjoy!

Nourishment: calories 30, fat 1, fiber 0.4, carbs 1, protein 0.1

Smooth Radishes

It's a smooth and delicious Keto veggie dish!
 Cook time: 10 minutes Cooking time: 25 minutes Servings: 1

Ingredients:
- 7 ounces radishes, cut in equal parts
- 2 tablespoons sharp cream
- 2 bacon cuts
- 1 tablespoon green onion, hacked
- 1 tablespoon cheddar, ground
- Hot sauce to the taste
- Salt and dark pepper to the taste

Directions:

1. Put radishes into a pot, add water to cover, heat to the point of boiling finished medium warmth, cook them for 10 minutes, and channel.

2. Warmth up a skillet over medium-high warmth, add bacon, cook until it's fresh, move to paper towels, channel oil, disintegrate and leave aside.

3. Return skillet to medium warmth, add radishes, mix and sauté them for 7 minutes.

4. Add onion, salt, pepper, hot sauce, and sharp cream, mix and cook for 7 minutes more.

5. Move to a plate, top with disintegrated bacon and cheddar, and serve.

Relax and enjoy!

Nourishment: calories 340, fat 23, fiber 3, carbs 6, protein 15

Radish Soup

Gracious, my God! These preferences divine!
 Cook time: 10 minutes Cooking time: 20 minutes Servings: 4

Ingredients:

- 2 packs radishes, cut in quarters
- Salt and dark pepper to the taste
- 6 cups chicken stock
- 2 stems celery, hacked
- 3 tablespoons coconut oil
- 6 garlic cloves, minced
- 1 yellow onion, hacked

Directions:

1. Warmth up a pot with the oil over medium warmth, add onion, celery, garlic, mix and cook for 5 minutes.

2. Add radishes, stock, salt and pepper, mix, heat to the point of boiling, spread also, stew for 15 minutes.

3. Separation into soup bowls and serve. Relax and enjoy!

Nourishment: calories 120, fat 2, fiber 1, carbs 3, protein 10

Scrumptious Avocado Serving of mixed greens

That is hugely scrumptious and reviving!

Preparing time: 10 minutes Cooking time: 0 minutes Servings: 4

Ingredients:
- 2 avocados, pitted and pounded
- Salt and dark pepper to the taste
- ¼ teaspoon lemon stevia
- 1 tablespoon white vinegar
- 14 ounces coleslaw blend
- Juice from 2 limes
- ¼ cup red onion, hacked
- ¼ cup cilantro, hacked
- 2 tablespoons olive oil

Directions:
1. Put coleslaw blend in a plate of mixed greens bowl. Add avocado crush and onions and throw to cover.
2. In a bowl, blend lime juice with salt, pepper, oil, vinegar, and stevia and mix well.
3. Add this to a plate of mixed greens, throw to cover, sprinkle cilantro, and serve.
Relax and enjoy!
Nourishment: calories 100, fat 10, fiber 2, carbs 5, protein 8

Avocado And Egg Serving of mixed greens

You will make it again, without a doubt!
Preparing time: 10 minutes Cooking time: 7 minutes Servings: 4

Ingredients:
- 4 cups blended lettuce leaves, torn
- 4 eggs
- 1 avocado, hollowed and cut
- ¼ cup mayonnaise
- 2 teaspoons mustard
- 2 garlic cloves, minced
- 1 tablespoon chives, cleaved
- Salt and dark pepper to the taste

Directions:
1. Place water in a pot, add some salt, add eggs, heat to the point of boiling finished medium-high warmth, bubble for 7 minutes, channel, cool, strip, and hack them.
2. In a plate of mixed greens bowl, blend lettuce in with eggs and avocado.
3. Add chives and garlic, some salt and pepper, and throw to cover.

4. In a bowl, blend mustard with mayo, salt, and pepper and mix well.
5. Add this to a plate of mixed greens, throw well, and serve immediately.
Relax and enjoy!
Nourishment: calories 234, fat 12, fiber 4, carbs 7, protein 12

Avocado And Cucumber Plate of mixed greens

You will request more! It's such a delicious summer serving of mixed greens!
 Preparing time: 10 minutes Cooking time: 0 minutes Servings: 4

Ingredients:
- 1 little red onion, cut
- 1 cucumber, cut
- 2 avocados, hollowed, stripped, and cleaved
- 1 pound cherry tomatoes, split
- 2 tablespoons olive oil
- ¼ cup cilantro, cleaved
- 2 tablespoons lemon juice
- Salt and dark pepper to the taste

Directions:
1. In a plate of mixed greens bowl, blend tomatoes in with cucumber, onion, and avocado and mix.
2. Add oil, salt, pepper, and lemon squeeze and throw to cover well.
3. Serve cold with cilantro on top.
Relax and enjoy!
Nourishment: calories 140, fat 4, fiber 2, carbs 4, protein 5

Tasty Avocado Soup

You will venerate this wonderful and tasty Keto soup!
 Cook time: 10 minutes Cooking time: 10 minutes Servings: 4

Ingredients:
- 2 avocados, hollowed, stripped, and hacked
- 3 cups chicken stock
- 2 scallions, cleaved
- Salt and dark pepper to the taste
- 2 tablespoons ghee
- 2/3 cup hefty cream

Directions:
1. Warmth up a pot with the ghee over medium warmth, add scallions, mix and cook for 2 minutes.
2. Add two and ½ cups stock, mix, and stew for 3 minutes.
3. In your blender, blend avocados in with the remainder of the stock, salt, pepper, and substantial cream, and heartbeat well.
4. Add this to the pot, mix well, cook for 2 minutes, and season with more salt and pepper.
5. Mix well, scoop into soup bowls and serve. Relax and enjoy!
Nourishment: calories 332, fat 23, fiber 4, carbs 6, protein 6

Heavenly Avocado and Bacon Soup

Have you ever caught wind of such a delectable Keto soup? At that point, it's time you find out additional about it!

Cook time: 10 minutes Cooking time: 10 minutes Servings: 4

Ingredients:
- 2 avocados, hollowed and cut in equal parts
- 4 cups chicken stock
- 1/3 cup cilantro, hacked
- Juice of ½ lime
- 1 teaspoon garlic powder
- ½ pound bacon, cooked and hacked
- Salt and dark pepper to the taste

Directions:
1. Put confidence in a pot and heat to the point of boiling over medium-high warmth.
2. In your blender, blend avocados with garlic powder, cilantro, lime squeeze, salt, and pepper and mix well.
3. Add this to stock and mix utilizing an inundation blender.
4. Add bacon, salt, pepper the taste, mix, cook for 3 minutes, and spoon into soup bowls and serve.

Relax and enjoy!

Nourishment: calories 300, fat 23, fiber 5, carbs 6, protein 17

Thai Avocado Soup

That is an incredible and fascinating soup!
Cooking time: 10 minutes Servings: 4

Ingredients:

- 1 cup of coconut milk
- 2 teaspoons Thai green curry glue
- 1 avocado, hollowed, stripped, and hacked
- 1 tablespoon cilantro, hacked
- Salt and dark pepper to the taste
- 2 cups veggie stock
- Lime wedges for serving

Directions:

1. In your blender, blend avocado with salt, pepper, curry glue, and coconut milk and heartbeat well.
2. Move this to a pot and warm up over medium warmth.
3. Add stock, mix, bring to a stew, and cook for 5 minutes.
4. Add cilantro, more salt, and pepper, mix, cook for one moment more, scoop into soup bowls, and present with lime wedges on the side.

Relax and enjoy!
Nourishment: calories 240, fat 4, fiber 2, carbs 6, protein 12

Basic Arugula Serving of mixed greens

It's light and incredibly delicious! Attempt it for supper!

Preparing time: 10 minutes Cooking time: 0 minutes Servings: 4

Ingredients:
- 1 white onion, slashed
- 1 tablespoon vinegar
- 1 cup boiling water
- 1 bundle infant arugula
- ¼ cup pecans, slashed
- 2 tablespoons cilantro, slashed
- 2 garlic cloves, minced
- 2 tablespoons olive oil
- Salt and dark pepper to the taste
- 1 tablespoon lemon juice

Directions:

1. In a bowl, blend water in with vinegar, add onion, leave aside for 5 minutes, channel well, and press.
2. Serving of mixed greens bowl, blend arugula in with pecans and onion and mix.
3. Add garlic, salt, pepper, lemon juice, cilantro, and oil, throw well also, serve. Relax and enjoy!
Nourishment: calories 200, fat 2, fiber 1, carbs 5, protein 7

Arugula Soup

You need to attempt this incredible Keto soup when you can!
 Preparing time: 10 minutes Cooking time: 13 minutes Servings: 6
Ingredients:
• 1 yellow onion, hacked
• 1 tablespoon olive oil
• 2 garlic cloves, minced
• ½ cup of coconut milk
• 10 ounces child arugula
• ¼ cup blended mint, tarragon, and parsley
• 2 tablespoons chives, hacked

- 4 tablespoons coconut milk yogurt
- 6 cups chicken stock
- Salt and dark pepper to the taste

Directions:

1. Warmth up a pot with the oil over medium-high warmth, add onion also, garlic, mix and cook for 5 minutes.
2. Add stock and milk, mix and bring to a stew.
3. Add arugula, tarragon, parsley, mint, mix, and cook everything for 6 minutes.
4. Add coconut yogurt, salt, pepper, chives, mix, cook for 2 minutes, partition into soup bowls, and serve.

Relax and enjoy!

Nourishment: calories 200, fat 4, fiber 2, carbs 6, protein 10

Arugula and Broccoli Soup

It's one of our number one soups!
Cook time: 10 minutes Cooking time: 20 minutes Servings: 4

Ingredients:

- 1 little yellow onion, hacked

- 1 tablespoon olive oil
- 1 garlic clove, minced
- 1 broccoli head, florets isolated
- Salt and dark pepper to the taste
- 2 and ½ cups veggie stock
- 1 teaspoon cumin, ground
- Juice of ½ lemon
- 1 cup arugula leaves

Directions:

1. Warmth up a pot with the oil over medium-high warmth, add onions, mix and cook for 4 minutes.

2. Add garlic, mix, and cook for one moment.

3. Add broccoli, cumin, salt, pepper, mix, and cook for 4 minutes.

4. Add stock, mix, and cook for 8 minutes.

5. Mix soup utilizing a drenching blender, add half of the arugula, and mix once more.

6. Add the remainder of the arugula, mix, and warmth up the soup once more.

7. Add lemon juice, mix, spoon into soup bowls and serve.

Relax and enjoy!

Nourishment: calories 150, fat 3, fiber 1, carbs 3, protein 7

Flavorful Zucchini Cream

That is a Keto comfort food you will Relax and enjoy without a doubt!
 Cook time: 10 minutes Cooking time: 25 minutes Servings: 8

Ingredients:
- 6 zucchinis, cut in equal parts and afterward cut
- Salt and dark pepper to the taste
- 1 tablespoon ghee
- 28 ounces veggie stock
- 1 teaspoon oregano, dried
- ½ cup yellow onion slashed
- 3 garlic cloves, minced
- 2 ounces parmesan, ground
- ¾ cup weighty cream

Directions:
1. Warmth up a pot with the ghee over medium-high warmth, add onion, mix and cook for 4 minutes.
2. Add garlic, mix, and cook for 2 minutes more.
3. Add zucchinis, mix, and cook for 3 minutes.

4. Add stock, mix, heat to the point of boiling, and stew over medium warmth for 15 minutes.
5. Add oregano, salt, and pepper, mix, take off warmth, and mix utilizing a submersion blender.
6. Warmth up soup once more, add hefty cream, mix and bring to a stew.
7. Add parmesan, mix, take off warmth, spoon into bowls, and serve immediately.
Relax and enjoy!
Nourishment: calories 160, fat 4, fiber 2, carbs 4, protein 8

Zucchini and Avocado Soup

This NOCARB soup is loaded with delicious ingredients and sound components!
 Cook time: 10 minutes Cooking time: 15 minutes Servings: 4

Ingredients:
• 1 major avocado, hollowed, stripped, and hacked
• 4 scallions, hacked
• 1 teaspoon ginger, ground
• 2 tablespoons avocado oil

- Salt and dark pepper to the taste
- 2 zucchinis, hacked
- 29 ounces veggie stock
- 1 garlic clove, minced
- 1 cup of water
- 1 tablespoon lemon juice
- 1 red chime pepper, cleaved

Directions:

1. Warmth up a pot with the oil over medium warmth, add onions, mix, what's more, cook for 3 minutes.

2. Add garlic and ginger, mix and cook for one moment.

3. Add zucchini, salt, pepper, water, and stock, mix, heat to the point of boiling, spread pot, and cook for 10 minutes.

4. Take off warmth, leave soup aside for several minutes, add avocado, mix, mix everything utilizing a drenching blender also, heat up once more.

5. Add more salt and pepper, chime pepper, lemon juice, mix, heat soup once more, scoop into soup bowls, and serve.

Relax and enjoy!

Nourishment: calories 154, fat 12, fiber 3, carbs 5, protein 4

Swiss chard Pie

You will consistently recollect this exquisite taste!
 Preparing time: 10 minutes Cooking time: 45 minutes Servings: 12

Ingredients:
• 8 cups Swiss chard, slashed
• ½ cup onion slashed
• 1 tablespoon olive oil
• 1 garlic clove, minced
• Salt and dark pepper to the taste
• 3 eggs
• 2 cups ricotta cheddar
• 1 cup mozzarella, destroyed
• A spot of nutmeg
• ¼ cup parmesan, ground
• 1 pound frankfurter, slashed

Directions:
1. Warmth up a skillet with the oil over medium warmth, add onions and garlic, mix and cook for 3 minutes.

2. Add Swiss chard, mix and cook for 5 minutes more.

3. Add salt, pepper, and nutmeg, mix, take off warmth and leave aside for a couple of moments.

4. In a bowl, whisk eggs with mozzarella, parmesan, and ricotta; furthermore, mix well.

5. Add Swiss chard blend and mix well.

6. Spread frankfurter meat on the lower part of a pie dish and press well.

7. Add Swiss chard and eggs blend, spread well, present in the stove at 350 degrees F, and heat for 35 minutes.

8. Leave pie aside to chill off, cut, and serve it. Relax and enjoy!

Nourishment: calories 332, fat 23, fiber 3, carbs 4, protein 23

Swiss Chard Plate of mixed greens

This plate of mixed greens is ideal for a quick supper!

Cook time: 10 minutes Cooking time: 20 minutes Servings: 4

Ingredients:
- 1 pack, Swiss chard, cut into strips
- 2 tablespoons avocado oil
- 1 little yellow onion, hacked
- A touch of red pepper pieces
- ¼ cup pine nuts, toasted
- ¼ cup raisins
- 1 tablespoon balsamic vinegar
- Salt and dark pepper to the taste

Directions:
1. Warmth up a dish with the oil over medium warmth, add chard and onions, mix and cook for 5 minutes.
2. Add salt, pepper, and pepper chips, mix and cook for 3 minutes more.
3. Put raisins in a bowl, add water to cover them, heat them in your microwave for one moment, leave aside for 5 minutes, and channel them well.
4. Add raisins and pine nuts to the dish, add vinegar, mix, cook for 3 minutes more, and partition among plates and serve.
Relax and enjoy!

Nourishment: calories 120, fat 2, fiber 1, carbs 4, protein 8

Green Serving of mixed greens

You should attempt this Keto serving of mixed greens!
 Preparing time: 10 minutes Cooking time: 0 minutes Servings: 4

Ingredients:
• 4 modest bunches grapes, divided
• 1 bundle Swiss chard, cleaved
• 1 avocado, hollowed, stripped, and cubed
• Salt and dark pepper to the taste
• 2 tablespoons avocado oil
• 1 tablespoon mustard
• 7 sage leaves, slashed
• 1 garlic clove, minced

Directions:
1. Serving of mixed greens bowl, blend Swiss chard in with grapes and avocado 3D shapes.
2. In a bowl, blend mustard in with the oil, sage, garlic, salt, and pepper also, whisk well.
3. Add this to a plate of mixed greens, throw to cover well, and serve.

Relax and enjoy!
Nourishment: calories 120, fat 2, fiber 1, carbs 4, protein 5

Catalan Style Greens

This veggie dish merely is extraordinary!
 Cook time: 10 minutes Cooking time: 15 minutes Servings: 4

Ingredients:
• 1 apple, cored and cleaved
• 1 yellow onion, cut
• 3 tablespoons avocado oil
• ¼ cup raisins
• 6 garlic cloves, cleaved
• ¼ cup pine nuts, toasted
• ¼ cup balsamic vinegar
• 5 cups blended spinach and chard
• Salt and dark pepper to the taste
• A touch of nutmeg

Directions:
1. Warmth up a container with the oil over medium-high warmth, add onion, mix and cook for 3 minutes.

2. Add apple, mix, and cook for 4 minutes more.

3. Add garlic, mix, and cook for one moment.

4. Add raisins, vinegar, and blended spinach and chard, mix, and cook for 5 minutes.

5. Add nutmeg, salt, and pepper, mix, cook for a couple of moments more, partition among plates, and serve.

Relax and enjoy!

Nourishment: calories 120, fat 1, fiber 2, carbs 3, protein 6

Swiss chard Soup

That is generous and rich!

Preparing time: 10 minutes Cooking time: 35 minutes Servings: 12

Ingredients:
- 4 cups Swiss chard, cleaved
- 4 cups chicken bosom, cooked and destroyed
- 2 cups water
- 1 cup mushrooms, cut
- 1 tablespoon garlic, minced
- 1 tablespoon coconut oil, liquefied
- ¼ cup onion, cleaved

- 8 cups chicken stock
- 2 cups yellow squash, cleaved
- 1 cup green beans, cut into medium pieces
- 2 tablespoons vinegar
- ¼ cup basil, hacked
- Salt and dark pepper to the taste
- 4 bacon cuts, hacked
- ¼ cup sundried tomatoes, hacked

Directions:

1. Warmth up a pot with the oil over medium-high warmth, add bacon, mix and cook for 2 minutes. Add tomatoes, garlic, onions, and mushrooms, mix and cook for 5 minutes.

2. Add water, stock and chicken, mix, and cook for 15 minutes.

3. Add Swiss chard, green beans, squash, salt, and pepper, mix and cook for 10 minutes more.

4. Add vinegar, basil, salt, and pepper if necessary, mix, spoon into soup bowls and serve.

Relax and enjoy!

Nourishment: calories 140, fat 4, fiber 2, carbs 4, protein 18

Unique Swiss chard Soup

It is so astonishing!
 Preparing time: 10 minutes Cooking time: 2 hours and 10 minutes Servings: 4
Ingredients:
- 1 red onion, hacked
- 1 pack, Swiss chard, cleaved
- 1 yellow squash, hacked
- 1 zucchini, hacked
- 1 green chime pepper, cleaved
- Salt and dark pepper to the taste
- 6 carrots, hacked
- 4 cups tomatoes, hacked
- 1 cup cauliflower florets, hacked
- 1 cup green beans, hacked
- 6 cups chicken stock
- 7 ounces canned tomato glue
- 2 cups water
- 1 pound hotdog, cleaved
- 2 garlic cloves, minced
- 2 teaspoons thyme, hacked
- 1 teaspoon rosemary, dried
- 1 tablespoon fennel, minced

- ½ teaspoon red pepper chips
- Some ground parmesan for serving

Directions:

1. Warmth up a skillet over medium-high warmth, add frankfurter and garlic, mix and cook until it earthy colors and move alongside its juices to your moderate cooker.

2. Add onion, Swiss chard, squash, ringer pepper, zucchini, carrots, tomatoes, cauliflower, green beans, tomato glue, stock, water, thyme, fennel, rosemary, pepper drops, salt and pepper, mix, spread, and cook on High for 2 hours.

3. Reveal pot, mix soup, scoop into bowls, sprinkle parmesan on top, and serve.

Relax and enjoy!

Nourishment: calories 150, fat 8, fiber 2, carbs 4, protein 9

Simmered Tomato Cream

It will fill your heart with joy much simpler!
Preparing time: 10 minutes Cooking time: 1-hour Servings: 8

Ingredients:
- 1 jalapeno pepper, slashed
- 4 garlic cloves, minced
- 2 pounds cherry tomatoes, cut in equal parts
- 1 yellow onion, cut into wedges
- Salt and dark pepper to the taste
- ¼ cup olive oil
- ½ teaspoon oregano, dried
- 4 cups chicken stock
- ¼ cup basil, cleaved
- ½ cup parmesan, ground

Directions:
1. Spread tomatoes and onion in a heating dish. Add garlic and bean stew pepper, season with salt, pepper, and oregano, and sprinkle the oil.
2. Throw to cover and heat in the broiler at 425 degrees F for 30 minutes.
3. Remove tomatoes blend from the broiler, move to a pot, add stock what's more, heat everything up over medium-high warmth.
4. Heat to the point of boiling, spread pot, diminish warmth, and stew for 20 minutes.

5. Mix utilizing a submersion blender, add salt and pepper to the taste and basil, mix and scoop into soup bowls.
6. Sprinkle parmesan on top and serve.
Relax and enjoy!
Nourishment: calories 140, fat 2, fiber 2, carbs 5, protein 8

Eggplant Soup

That is what you required today!
Cook time: 10 minutes Cooking time: 50 minutes Servings: 4

Ingredients:
• 4 tomatoes
• 1 teaspoon garlic, minced
• ¼ yellow onion, cleaved
• Salt and dark pepper to the taste
• 2 cups chicken stock
• 1 straight leaf
• ½ cup hefty cream
• 2 tablespoons basil, cleaved
• 4 tablespoons parmesan, ground
• 1 tablespoon olive oil
• 1 eggplant, cleaved

Directions:
1. Spread eggplant pieces on a heating sheet, blend in with the oil, onion, garlic, salt, and pepper, present in the broiler at 400 degrees F furthermore, heat for 15 minutes.
2. Put water in a pot, heat to the point of boiling over medium warmth, add tomatoes, steam them for 1 minute, strip them and slash.
3. Remove eggplant blend from the broiler and move to a pot.
4. Add tomatoes, stock, narrows leaf, salt, and pepper, mix, bring to a bubble, and stew for 30 minutes.
5. Add heavy cream, basil, and parmesan, mix, scoop into soup bowls, and serve.
Relax and enjoy!
Nourishment: calories 180, fat 2, fiber 3, carbs 5, protein 10

Eggplant Stew

That is ideal for a family meal!
Cook time: 10 minutes Cooking time: 30 minutes Servings: 4
Ingredients:

- 1 red onion, slashed
- 2 garlic cloves, slashed
- 1 bundle parsley, cleaved
- Salt and dark pepper to the taste
- 1 teaspoon oregano, dried
- 2 eggplants, cut into medium lumps
- 2 tablespoons olive oil
- 2 tablespoons tricks, slashed
- 1 small bunch of green olives, hollowed and cut
- 5 tomatoes, hacked
- 3 tablespoons spice vinegar

Directions:

1. Warmth up a pot with the oil over medium warmth, add eggplant, oregano, salt, and pepper, mix and cook for 5 minutes.
2. Add garlic, onion, and parsley, mix and cook for 4 minutes.
3. Add tricks, olives, vinegar, tomatoes, mix, and cook for 15 minutes.
4. Mix more salt and pepper if necessary, mix, partition into bowls, and serve.

Relax and enjoy!

Nourishment: calories 200, fat 13, fiber 3, carbs 5, protein 7

Broiled Ringer Peppers Soup

That isn't merely tasty! It's Keto and reliable too!

Preparing time: 10 minutes Cooking time: 15 minutes Servings: 6

Ingredients:
- 12 ounces cooked ringer peppers, cleaved
- 2 tablespoons olive oil
- 2 garlic cloves, minced
- 29 ounces could chicken stock
- Salt and dark pepper to the taste
- 7 ounces water
- 2/3 cup hefty cream
- 1 yellow onion, cleaved
- ¼ cup parmesan, ground
- 2 celery stems, cleaved

Directions:
1. Warmth up a pot with the oil over medium warmth, add onion, garlic, celery, salt, pepper, mix, and cook for 8 minutes.
2. Add chime peppers, water, and stock, mix, heat to the point of boiling, spread, diminish warmth, and stew for 5 minutes.

3. Utilize a submersion blender to puree the soup; at that point, add more salt, pepper, and cream, mix, heat to the point of boiling, and take off warmth.
4. Spoon into bowls, sprinkle parmesan, and serve.
Relax and enjoy!
Nourishment: calories 176, fat 13, fiber 1, carbs 4, protein 6

Delectable Cabbage Soup

This delectable cabbage soup will turn into your new most loved soup indeed before long!
 Preparing time: 10 minutes Cooking time: 45 minutes Servings: 8
Ingredients:
• 1 garlic clove, minced
• 1 cabbage head, hacked
• 2 pounds meat, ground
• 1 yellow onion, hacked
• 1 teaspoon cumin
• 4 bouillon 3D squares
• Salt and dark pepper to the taste
• 10 ounces canned tomatoes and green chilies

• 4 cups water

Directions:

1. Warmth up a dish over medium warmth, add hamburger, mix, and earthy colored for a few moments.

2. Add onion, mix, cook for 4 minutes more and move to a pot.

3. Warmth up, add cabbage, cumin, garlic, bouillon shapes, tomatoes furthermore, chilies and water, mix, heat to the point of boiling over high warmth, spread, lessen temperature and cook for 40 minutes.

4. Season with salt and pepper, mix, scoop into soup bowls and serve.

Relax and enjoy!

Nourishment: calories 200, fat 3, fiber 2, carbs 6, protein 8

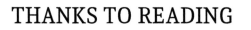
THANKS TO READING